Apple is not just a fruit. A cancer fighter: Amazing health benefits of apple

By

Mercy Obidake

Table of content

Introduction

Apple originated in the Middle East about 4000 years ago! It is one of the most popular fruit on earth. People who are health conscious have found the fruit highly rewarding. It is an indispensable fruit. It is highly medicinal and known for nutrition and health care.

Research has revealed that the nutrients contained in apple plays a major role in the promotion of human health in various ways.

Chapter One

History of Apple

In existence, one of the oldest varieties is the apple fruit. Research has shown that humans have enjoyed apples since 6500 B.C. Apple is among the favorite fruits of Romans and the Ancient Greeks.

The apple tree commonly called Malus domestica is a deciduous tree in the rose family known for its tasty, pomaceous fruit called apple. The tree originated in Central Asia, where Malus sieversii, its ancestor, is present till today. Apples have grown for thousands of years in Europe and Asia, and through the aid of the European colonists were brought to North America.

In many cultures, Apples have mythological and religious significance including Greek, Norse and European Christian traditions.

In so many religious traditions, apples appear as a forbidden or mystical fruit. In religion, folktales and mythology, the word "apple" was used as a generic term for foreign fruit, aside berries, as late as the 17th century.

In Greek mythology, as a part of his Twelve Labors,

the Greek hero Heracles was expected to travel to the Garden of the Hesperides and collect the golden apples off the Tree of Life.

Eris, the Greek goddess of discord, became angry after she was excluded from Peleus and Thetis wedding. In retaliation, she tossed a golden apple inscribed Καλλίστη, which means "For the most beautiful one" into the wedding party. Hera, Aphrodite and Athena, the three goddesses claimed the apple. The recipient was to be selected by the Paris of Troy. Hera and Athena both bribed him; Aphrodite on the other hand tempted him with the world's most beautiful woman, Helen of Sparta. Aphrodite was awarded the apple; this caused the Trojan War.

The apple became sacred to Aphrodite. Symbolically, to throw an apple at someone meant one's love; and similarly, catching it meant one's acceptance of that love. An epigram claiming authorship by Plato states in Christian art, Adam and Eve showcased the apple as a symbol of sin. Famous Christian tradition has held the opinion that it was an apple that Eve lured Adam to share with her.

Chapter Two

Health benefits of apple

Apples contain several health benefits. They are listed below:

*** It contains several nutrients which makes it highly nutritious for the body.**
A medium sized apple contains the following nutrients:
* 25 grams of carbs
*95 grams of calorie
*6% of the RDI in potassium
*4 grams of fiber
*5% of vitamin C RDI
*14% of vitamin C RDI
*About 4% of the RDI in magnesium, copper and vitamins A, E, B1, B2 and B6

Several health benefits are a result of these compounds. An apple's skin contains polyphenols and fibre. A good source of fiber and vitamin C is apple. They also contain polyphenols, which has a lot of health benefits.

*** It aids in weight Loss**

The water and fiber contained in apple, when consumed, can enable you get full quickly. In a research carried out, participants who ate few slices of apple before a meal felt much fuller than those who drank apple juice or other products.

In another research conducted, fifty overweight men added either apples or oat cookies to their diets for ten weeks. Each item had the same calorie and fiber content. Those who consumed the apples lost 2 lbs and consumed less calories overall.

Apples are energy-dense, and they contain natural compounds which aids weight loss.

*** It helps in the prevention of heart diseases.**

In researches carried out, apples have been linked to enabling a lower risk of heart disease. Soluble fiber is contained in apples, which helps to reduce the level of blood cholesterol.

Apples also contain Polyphenols. These nutrients

have antioxidant effects and they help in lowering blood pressure.

Apples promote heart health in several ways. They have a lot of soluble fiber, which helps in the reduction of cholesterol and polyphenols, which lower blood pressure and the risk of having stroke.

The health benefits of apple just cannot be over emphasized.

* It fights against constipation and diarrhea

Apples contain fiber which fights against constipation and diarrhea. Fiber absorbs excess water from your stool in order to slow down your bowels.

* It neutralizes irritable bowel syndrome

Doctors recommend a high intake of fiber in your diet and less consumption of fatty and dairy foods to avoid irritable bowel syndrome, it is a good thing that Apple contains fiber.

* It averts hemorrhoids

Much pressure in the rectal and pelvic areas can cause hemorrhoids. Apple contains fiber which helps to protect against hemorrhoid by preventing you from excessive strain in the bathroom.

* It lowers the risk of diabetes

Apples contain polyphenols which help to prevent tissue damage to beta cells in the pancreas. The body's insulin is produced by beta cells. People with type 2 diabetes often have damaged beta cells.

A great health benefit of apple is its ability to lower the risk of diabetes. Health benefits of apple are indeed obvious.

* It promotes good gut bacteria

The pectin in apple feeds the good bacteria in your gut. Fiber is not absorbed by your intestine during digestion; instead, it goes to the colon, where good bacteria growth is promoted.

Good bacteria's are being fed by the fiber in apple; this enables protection against obesity, type 2 heart disease and diabetes.

* It prevent cataracts

Apples contain antioxidants which help to prevent the development of cataract.

* It gives healthier and whiter teeth

Chewing and biting an apple stimulates saliva production in the mouth which reduces tooth decay by reducing bacteria levels. For healthier teeth, try chewing more apples.

* It prevents Parkinson disease

People who consume fruits or foods rich in fiber gain a great amount of protection against Parkinson's disease. Scientists have come to a conclusion that this is as a result of the radical-fighting power of the antioxidants in apple.

* It prevents cancer

Apple lowers the risk of cancer. It contains compounds that fight cancer. Apples provide antioxidant and anti-inflammatory effects in the body.

* It fights Asthma

Apples are rich in Antioxidant which protects the lungs from oxidative damages. Quercetin is a flavonoid found in the skin of the apple. It aids in the regulation of the immune system and also reduces inflammation. Apples contain anti-inflammatory compounds and antioxidant which helps in the regulation of immune responses and also fights against asthma.

A great health benefit of apple is its ability to fight asthma.

* A good health of the bone

Research conducted has revealed that the anti-inflammatory compounds and antioxidant in apple helps in promoting bone strength density.

Also, bone mass as you grow older in age can be preserved by eating lots of apple.

* It prevents stomach injury from NSAIDs

Non-steroidal anti-inflammatory drugs (NSAIDs) can cause great damage to the stomach lining.

A study conducted in rats found that freeze-dried apple extract helps in protecting stomach cells from injury as a result of NSAIDs. Catechin and chlorogenic acid in apples are two compounds which were helpful.

The compounds in apple help to protect the stomach lining from injury as a result of NSAID painkillers.

The health benefit of apple is also obvious in its ability to protect the stomach lining of the body from injury.

* It protects the brain in old age

The juice gotten from apple has great health advantages for age-related mental decline. The juice of apple helps in the preservation of acetylcholine, which reduces with age. Acetylcholine in low level can result in Alzheimer's disease. Whole apples also contain the same compounds in apple juice. However, eating the whole apple is healthier.

Chapter Three

Harvestings

The following factors determine the harvesting time of apple:

* Color
*Firmness
*Ease of picking

The longevity of apples is determined by the proper time of picking and accurate storage. The harvesting of apples simply depends on the climatic conditions and bloom time of the tree during the budding season. Maturity of the fruit can be delayed by certain factors, such as cool conditions, cloudy or drought conditions. It is proper to harvest home-grown apples when they reach minimum maturity but are not fully ripe. At minimum maturity period the apples are usually firm and crisp. The quality of the fruit can be preserved by proper storage-by ripening slowly and reducing water loss.

Chapter Four

Varieties of Apple

Ananasrenette

Ananas Reinette means "royal pineapple" When translated in English. It is round and symmetrical in shape. The fruit has a yellowish- white flesh which is juicy and crunchy.

Arkansas Black

It has a flattened shape with a dark red color. When stored, the skin continues to darken. Amongst apple cultivars, it is the darkest in color. Arkansas Black apple has an intense aromatic flavor.

Bonza

It has an odd shape with a semi-sweet taste. It can be eaten raw or used for apple butter or apple sauce.

Braeburn

It has a crispy and spicy-sweet flavor which distinguishes it from other apple. Breaburn apple has a glossy skin, striped red blush over yellow.

Bramley

It has a sour taste, which is enjoyed when cooked. It becomes fluffy and golden when cooked.

Fuji It has a mild delicious flavor, often large in size and incredibly great for cooking. Its color is a lovely pink speckled flush on top of a yellow-green background.

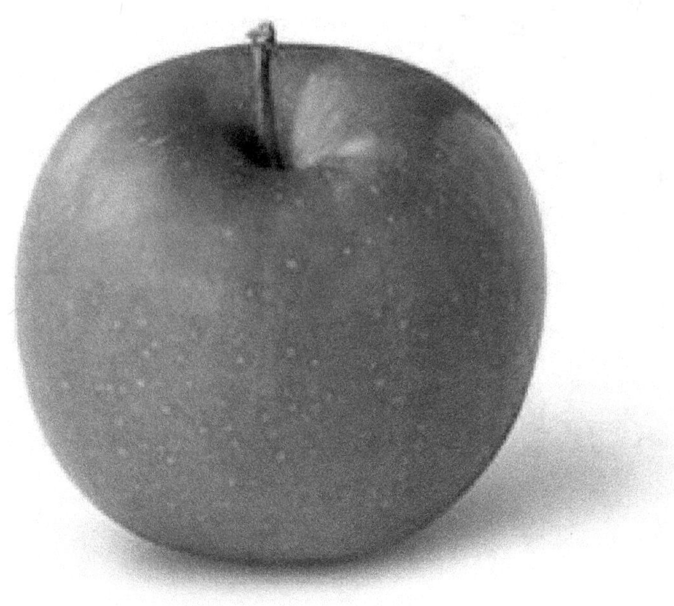

Gala

It has a lovely red sheen with bright-yellow

undertones. It is very rich in dietary fiber.

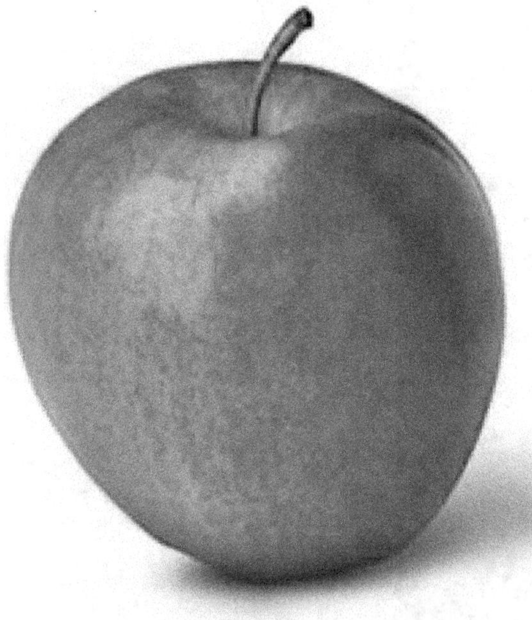

Golden delicious

It is one of the most vital apple varieties. When cooked or baked, a rich mild flavor exudes out of it.

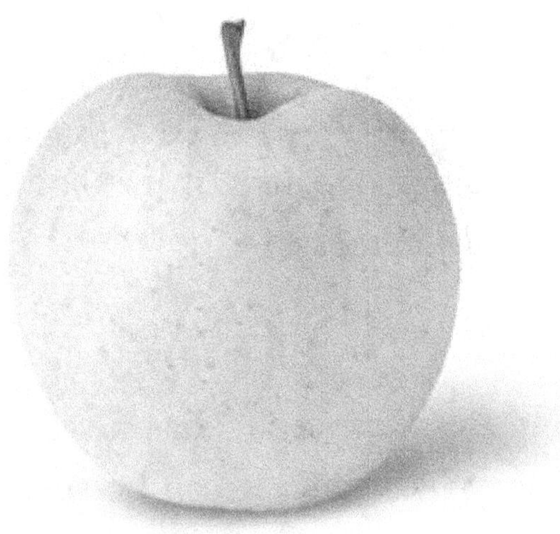

Goldrenette

It has a greenish-yellow to orange skin color streaked with red tinge. Mostly preferred when it is cooked to eating it raw or making sauce.

Granny smith

It can be used in salads. It has a very sharp "acidic" taste.

Jonagold

Its gleaming white flesh gives a delicious flavor.

Jonathan

It can be eaten fresh or used for processing. It blends well in sauces and cider because of its slight spicy flavor and exceptional juiciness.

Lobo

It can be used in making desserts. Lobo has a semi acidic, sweet, bit strawberry-like taste. It can be seen during the mid September.

McIntosh

It has a creamy flesh which makes it good for apple sauce or apple butter. It has a simple and aromatic flavor.

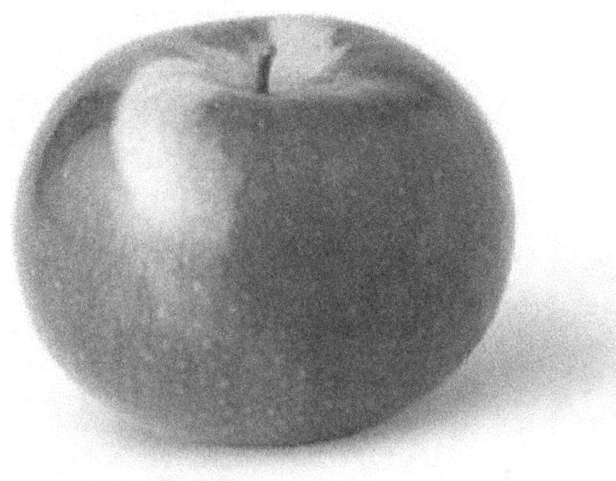

Pacific rose

It has a rose-pink color, with a delicious, refreshing and crispy taste. It can be harvested in April.

Cripps pink

Grown under particular conditions, they are great for salads, sauce, snacks, baking, pies and freezing.

Red delicious apple

It has a conical shape with a lovely aromatic flavor. Its color is bright red. It is best for making salads and snacking.

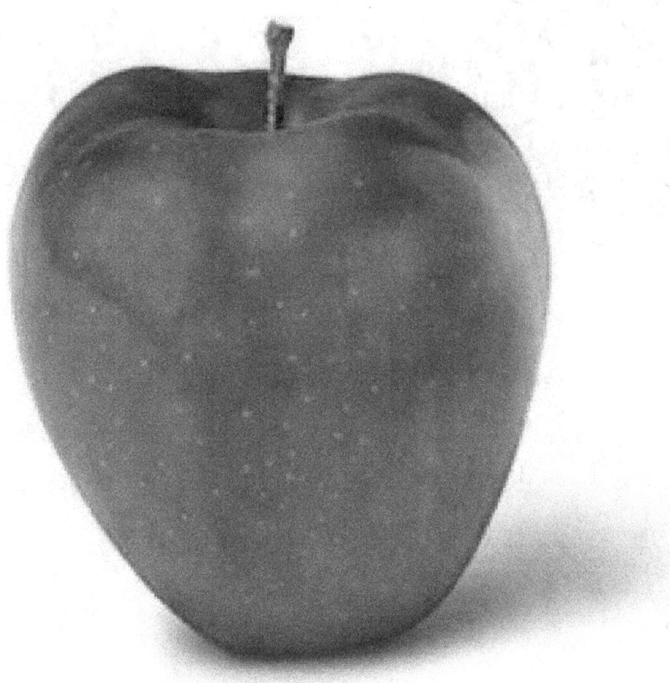

Yellow Transparent

It has a juicy sharp taste and sweet flavor, good for freezing, drying, juice, sauce and wine. It is a very good apple for cooking.

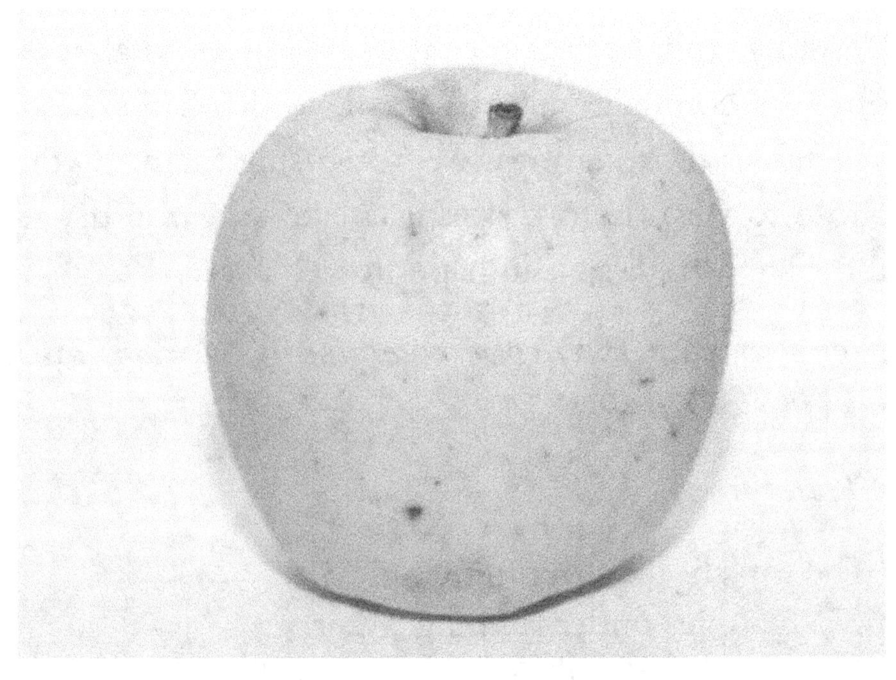

Chapter Five

Cleansing, storage and serving Tips

Fresh fruits are an important part of a healthy diet.

Washing fruits as it is meant to be is very vital, it is often recommended to wash your fruits and vegetables thoroughly just before using them. If you chose to wash before storing, make sure you dry it thoroughly with a clean paper towel.

Steps to take for proper cleansing, storage and serving of Apples

Cleansing:

*The top should be trimmed off.
*Wash apples under running water.
*Get rid of waxy preservative by scrubbing it.
*Cut the ends of the stems before eating.

Serving

*The skin contains most of the fiber, so it is best to eat it with its peel.

Apples when cut and exposed to air turn brownish in color. When sliced, ensure that you rinse in water containing some drops of lemon before serving.

When diced, serve with yogurts, ice-cream, cereals, confectioneries, etc,
Apple cubes can be added to fresh salads.

Conclusion

Apple is a nutritious fruit. The various health benefits of apple cannot be over emphasized. Regular intake of apple protects against excess weight gain, heart disease, cancer, diabetes, hemorrhoids, memory loss, Parkinson disease, asthma, stroke, constipation, etc.

Get an Apple today. It is not just a fruit. It is so much more.

ABOUT THE AUTHOR

Mercy Obidake is a Writer, TV presenter, and blogger. She writes scripts for movies and Television programs, novels, articles and eBooks.

Aside from writing, she enjoys providing humanitarian services to the less privileged in society.